Overcoming Depression

The steps I took to win the fight.

Table of Contents

1: Acknowledge you suffer from it..4

2: Accept that you don't want to live your life with depression..7

3: Take notes of the situations that trigger your depression and which ones take you away from it................9

4: Once you start to determine step 3, focus on avoiding the situations that triggers your depression.........12

5: Don't say "I (you) can't" 16

6: Every day, do your best to embrace the situation(s) that makes you happier...20

7: Pay attention to what you eat...22

8: Be very careful if you drink alcohol or smoke weed........25

9: Pay attention to the company you keep..........................28

10: Remember the key to winning the war? 31

11: Be careful with pills!..32

12: There is always someone who cares!!!.......................34

13: Start working on your passion..36

14: Choose your music wisely..38

15: Do as much as you can while you can…………………………40

16: The present is a gift…………………………………………………45

17: Exercise. Get back to nature……………………………………47

18: Final thoughts……………………………………………………50

Acknowledge You Suffer From It.

Depression is a disorder that puts you in a mode of sadness and a general loss of interest. We all have our bad days and good days, days on which we are full of joy and energy, days we are sad and with no desire to even move.

To win the war on depression, we must first acknowledge that we suffer from it. Sometimes we feel that if we ignore it long enough it will just go away, when in reality it does not. It is doing the opposite and will continue to build. Ignoring depression can be visualized as sweeping dirt under the rug; every time you ignore, you sweep it under, then, as time goes on, that dirt builds up becoming larger and larger, and begins to show with uneven surfaces above. Same with our lives, it will only be a matter of time before ignoring it takes a toll and before you know it, you're locked in your room, no motivation to leave, talking yourself into low self-esteem, ignoring family and friends who love us dearly, and the list goes on.

The earlier you accept the reality that you are suffering, the sooner you can start taking steps to gain control of your life and feelings. I remember the day I chose to accept my reality and changed my fate. I was home on my native island after being sent back by the Canadian Immigration, while waiting for my paperwork to be processed. I laid in my room for weeks with no motivation to even step outside my bedroom "cell" that I had locked myself into, only coming out to eat and use the bathroom. My mom would always be checking up on me and asking, "why don't you go to the beach or out with your friends?". I kept saying that nothing was wrong, and the time will soon pass, and all will be well! What started as days quickly turned into weeks and weeks into months. By the middle of the third month, I realized that I was out of cash, with no silver lining of when the immigration paperwork would be completed. I started noticing that my mom was becoming increasingly worried about me. It was then reality was accepted. I had waded myself into a pit of depression and needed to dig myself out. For the next few days, I went from "playing dead" to planning and executing how I was going to get my life back and these are the steps that helped me:

Nathaniel Branden said *"The first step toward change is awareness. The second step is acceptance".*

Accept That You Don't Want To Live Your Life With Depression.

Acknowledging that you suffer from it is one thing, but unless you come to terms with yourself and be forthright that you do not wish to live another day being sad and depressed then you must make it known that your journey to fight depression has officially begun.

Start by trying to remember the last time or phase in your life where you felt genuinely happy or where you were "unstoppable" in accomplishing what you wanted to. Remember the joy and freedom you felt in those times. If the memories are short lived and can't be grasped, then envision what "freedom" means to you and what your life/lifestyle will be with that freedom. With the vision now in your head, keep it as your highest pedestal in life, kind of like "the carrot held in front of the donkey to get it where you want it to go". This vision is to be kept "on" your mind as much as possible and should bring a smile to your face each time, knowing that the feeling will be great when you regain your freedom and break the shackles of depression.

I simply laid in my bed as depressed as I was and thought of the days when I would go out with my friends and family just to socialize; I remembered it being so much FUN. I thought of how fun it was being on the beach, going sailing, bike riding and just being outdoors in general. Remembering the joy of those encounters brought me to tears of joy and that was basically when I accepted that I was done with being depressed. I wanted the fun back, I wanted to be happy again.

Nelson Mandela said, *"Speak what you seek until you see what you've said"*. Speak your victory into reality.

Take Notes Of The Situations That Trigger Your Depression And Which Ones Take You Away From It.

At this point in time, we are starting to make the baby steps towards victory. This step requires you to "live and let live." By this you are not to get wound up in feelings and are not to go "hunting" for answers. Go about the day in a normal day to day manner, don't try to fix anything in this phase, but pay attention to shifts in mood. If at any moment you find yourself feeling down and out of it, try to pinpoint the time where your feelings started to change and what was the situation surrounding it. The same thing goes if you're feeling jolly and full of life; is it when you're in a particular place? Is it when friends or family come around? Being by the ocean, working on cars, your job? Anything.

Once you notice a shift in your mood write it down. Make a note in a book or your phone that says something like:

1- I've noticed myself feeling very happy around 12:34 pm when I was at Xyz and Abc showed up.

2- I found myself feeling very down around 45:67am (I still have your attention), I was heading to MNOP to do this or that.

At the end of the day, look through your notes and review them carefully, was it someone or was it some place that brought about the shift in feelings? Was it a random thought that crossed your mind and triggered an upward or downward spiral? The more notes you have the more likely you are to pick up trends and start connecting dots.

The fact that I was back on my island when I embarked on this "adventure", most of my notes consisted of the places and situations that made me happy. The circumstances surrounding my overall depression was due to feeling "stranded" as I waited for my documents to be approved. In my spare time I would try to think back on situations in Canada that had triggered any of these reactions, making note of them in preparation for when I returned to Canada. I was armed and ready for the battles ahead.

Ralph Marston said "*Happiness is a choice, not a result. Nothing will make you happy until you choose to be happy*".

Once You Start To Determine Step 3, Focus On Avoiding The Situations That Triggers Your Depression.

We can do research and take all the notes in the world but unless we begin to act and execute accordingly, then those notes become a waste. After collecting and reviewing what triggers your moods, begin to come up with ways of avoiding what ignites your depression and gravitate towards what brings you joy. One of the biggest illusions being fed into today's world is, if we have a "good job", to stick with it no matter what. I remember a few years back; I had a job as head truck driver and the right-hand man for the boss. This job had me doing early mornings and late nights. I was also the one that most drivers reported to with queries they had, along with other incidents.

At first the pay felt great, and life felt "good" but then things started to take a turn down a slippery slope when the weight of my job requirements started to become more than I could handle mentally. The signs that stood out the most to me was that my "fuse" had become super short, I was quick to snap at everyone and anyone. When I arrived home after work at night, all it took was for my wife to say "hi" and I was ready to lose it. At work, people started to ease back slowly from being around me and chose very carefully what words they would say as I was increasingly becoming easily offended or irritated (keep in mind that at the start I was a jolly fella who always loved to help). As time went by it became conspicuous that this "new me" was taking a heavy toll on my family life and I decided enough was enough.

    I had made many mentions of leaving this job for the betterment of my mental health but quickly ran into doubts as I was being advised by my peers not to quit as I was making decent money and was also among the highest paid of the group at that time. Being counselled by my group and some co-workers, I decided to "stick it out". My symptoms continued to grow, my fuse got shorter and shorter, and my family life got more miserable. Until I said, "enough IS enough."

After parting from this job, it placed a huge dent in my financial situation, but created unimaginable growth in my mental wellbeing. I was back to smiling, helping, loving and had many moments of "stopping to smell the roses".

Though there were always trickle grapevine talks of me being crazy for quitting such a decent paying job; no one at the time but me and my family understood the relief I felt for my "freedom".

Steven Bartlett said *"Your mental health is more important than your career, money, other people's opinions, that event you said you would attend, your partners mood and your families wishes, combined. If taking care of yourself means letting someone down, then let someone down". Make your mental health your number one priority."*

Don't Say "I (you) Can't".

I cannot say this any simpler, or clearer! The beginning will always be the hardest part, pushing that big wheel to its first turn will always be extremely difficult. This is where many people throw in the towel before they even begin. Keep in mind that beating depression is not a race, it's not a competition, but there is a reward, your FREEDOM.

Sometimes to get ahead we must "unlearn" many things that may have caused this problem in the first place, then replace it with information more designed to suit your individual need(s). A famous Henry Ford quote reads, *"Whether you think you can, or you think you can't – you're right,"*. Keeping that in mind, there will be times where you'll find yourself in a predicament that makes choosing impossible. In the case of my job as mentioned earlier, I was facing "freedom," or the choice of a roof above my family's head and food on the table".

The world has taught us to forget freedom and live up to the "standard" that society teaches us, but I'm going to tell you this, never say you can't, never say you have no choice. I am not telling you to stop doing everything suddenly, some things you can stop immediately with little to no consequences, while others may require time and a transition period. If you find yourself hating your job but needing to keep on working to keep food on the table, don't say "I can't leave." Start looking for a new job or even request to move to another department if possible or find creative ways to make money so you can begin that transition. There have been times and times again where I told myself I can't beat this, I can't win depression, I must suck it up and bury this feeling and just do what I must to "survive," but I choose to make a stand against that and let it be known that <u>I CAN, and I WILL!</u> So, I quit. It was the best thing I ever did: BELIEVE.

Please take note that I'm not in any way pushing to say your job is the "problem." Personally, for me, I knew this was a major contributing factor and it weighed heavily on my life, so it's only natural for me to use it as an example.

Walter D. Wintle said *"If you think you are beaten, you are. If you think you dare not, you don't, if you like to win, but you think you can't, it is almost certain you won't. If you think you'll lose, you're lost out of the world we find, success begins with a fellow's will, it's all in the state of mind. If you think you are outclassed, you are. You've got to think high to rise, you've got to be sure of yourself before you can ever win a prize. Life's battle doesn't always go to the stronger or faster man, but sooner or later the man who wins is the man WHO THINKS HE CAN!".*

Every day, Do Your Best To Embrace The Situation(s) That Makes You Happier.

A major point to always remember is that fighting depression is like fighting a war, the key to winning the war is to focus on winning the small battles, you will win the war eventually. If you go about it trying to fight depression on a whole, you are likely to lose, instead, you are to focus on winning the battles one day at a time. Fighting the war head on is like taking a weed trimmer just to trim the top off the weed and every time it grows back, it comes with vengeance, thicker and stronger than before. While focusing on the battle, it is like getting down on your hands and knees with the focus on pulling the "root" out of the ground.

As the days go by, with the goal of "freedom" in mind, naturally you will lean towards staying in your happy zone and doing more and more to refrain from what triggers the negative effect. One day at a time, one foot in front the other, transition yourself from the negative causing effects and keep towards what brings you joy and happiness.

Rory Vaden said, *"Success is not owned; it is rented, and that rent is due everyday"*.

Pay Attention To What You EAT.

Food tends to fly under the radar and puts us in some very bad moods without being called out as the culprit. Research has shown that processed foods with lots of added sugar, salt, and fat, can be very likely linked to your depression and anxiety, this brings me to a famous phrase from the movie Austin Powers: "I eat because I'm unhappy, and I'm unhappy because I eat." This is a very vicious cycle that one may find themselves in. Many people have different reasons that may cause them to be in a depressive state. For some, it may be the people they are around, the place(s) they live, work, or visit, and for some it may just be as simple as their diet or a combination of all of these. The list goes on.

Many times, when working in a fast-paced environment, and long hours, we force ourself to eat and buy fast foods (processed foods) which can cause inflammation throughout the body and brain, which may contribute to mental disorders like depression and/or anxiety.

This is a list of foods that I have uncovered as major depression enhancers and culprits of my moody ways. I will suggest you cut back on your intake of, or avoid them all together if possible as most would likely cause you to be depressed and/or anxious:

- processed food
- fried food (most fast foods)
- candy
- pastries
- refined cereals (often have high levels of added sugar, fat, or salt)
- high fat dairy products, etc.

I then switched to having higher intakes of fruits, vegetables, and supplements rich in zinc, iron, Vitamins B and D, magnesium, omega 3, fiber-rich grains, and fish. These are stuff that I added to my diet that have worked greatly for me and helped maintain an uplifted mood. Please note I am in no shape or form a doctor and I'm only sharing what have worked for me in my diet, please use diligent research on what may or may not work for you and consult your doctor accordingly.

Anthelme Brillat-Savarin said *"You are what you eat",* a simple way I found to interpret this is: eat bad, look bad, feel bad, or eat good, look good, feel good.

Be Very Careful If You Drink Alcohol Or Smoke Weed.

Alcohol, weed or any other type of drug affects everyone differently, some may experience extremely good benefits while others may have catastrophic results. Any forms of mental relief from any type of drug are normally short lived, and upon leaving the body, the depression and/or anxiety cycle builds even higher than before, creating an ongoing cycle.

There was a time in my life when I drank and smoked heavily throughout my depression phase. During this time, I thought the alcohol was helping to take away my bad feelings and credited the alcohol with great praise for what it did. Then, every time I felt like my depression was coming back, I would run for another round of drinking just to drown out the feeling as much as possible. It wasn't until later in life when I decided to stop drinking and smoking for the sake of my liver, lungs, and everything else, that I realized how much trouble I was in for not dealing with my unresolved issues. As the substances began to withdraw from my body, I felt the world had now thrown me back into the battle zone. As I weathered the storm and time passed, I noticed a feeling like I was in a state of "natural high", like my depression had somehow eased. At this point I decided to put my newfound discovery to the test and be the "lab rat". I jumped heavily to alcohol and smoking for a short period of time then stopped. My speculation was correct as my depressive state came back like a wrecking ball and I would curl up in my sorrows until all the chemicals left my system, leaving me feeling free as a bird.

To this day I have limited my alcohol intake to 1-2 beers, and mostly just at social events as I noticed taking in large amounts would later trigger my depressive feelings. I use marijuana on very rare occasions (more on a medical basis) or if I'm having trouble sleeping for an extended period, or if I have no appetite. Other than that, I refrain from using as much as possible. I should also mention that I'm located in Canada where marijuana use is legal. (Use with discretion if really needed).

Shirley Anita Chisholm said, *"It's not drugs or alcohol that makes one an addict, it is the need to escape from a harsh reality"*.

Pay Attention To The Company You Keep.

Do you have friends or family who you grew up with, that have now developed characteristics that somehow seems to get on your nerves whenever they are around? You must put your mental wellbeing first and exclude yourself from their presence or limit your exposure to them. Learn to remove all toxic people from your life.

When I started to pay close attention to the situation(s) that triggered my depression, I could not help but notice that being around certain people made me feel very uneasy or uncomfortable. There is this one "friend" who comes to mind that I have always found myself being around and trying to share ideas and grow with. After a while, I noticed that every time I left their presence, I would feel drained, annoyed, sad, and any word you can think of to this nature. After embarking on my journey, I started paying close attention to the circumstances surrounding why I always felt the way I felt around them. It had caught my attention that no matter what I said or how I said it, my ideas were always shot down and met with doubts and no understanding. While on the flip side, any ideas shared with me was met with words or encouragement and support. I set out to figure out why they reacted that way in comparison to the way I do. After doing some research I came across two words: frequency and vibration. Upon learning these words, I went down the "rabbit hole" of YouTube and looked for any information I could find to gain knowledge of the topic. I have now learnt how to detect/spot low or high frequency in people, who I can get along with and who I can't, so now I save myself some trouble and stick with those of higher vibration.

Remember, we are here for your mental wellbeing, so I will advise you to not be afraid to stay away from any friends or family who makes you feel unwanted or uneasy in any way, no matter how difficult it may seem!

Khayal 'Aly said *"Now that you're awake, beware of the company you keep; some help you to rise, others tell you to go back to sleep. You've slept enough, now it's time for you to stay woke; read the Prophetic scriptures: the sublime words that they spoke. Seek knowledge and wisdom and discover perennial philosophy; you need spiritual science to uncover traditional theosophy. When you go deep in meditation you will manifest your real form; can you really go back to sleep if you were blessed to be reborn?"*.

Remember The Key To Winning The War?

Over time, your feelings may relapse repeatedly but following these steps should make the timespan less and less until you feel the freedom. As stated before, to win the war, we must shift the focus to winning smaller, daily battles one day at a time. Eventually, winning battles will become so constant and easy that before realizing it, you will already be crowned victor of the war of your mind.

Back to the steps.

Be Careful With Pills!

As the reality of the medical field states "A patient cured is a customer lost". It is sad to say or think of such but it's the reality of times. I have seen the bitter end of someone taking depression pills prescribed by their doctor and going against my advice not to take them, then plummeting so far into a depressive state, that it lead to suicidal thoughts and full withdrawal from kids and family, so much so that even I had a moment of believing that there was no coming back. As time passed, this person got a second opinion from another doctor and was told that they were not to abruptly stop the medication but instead slowly reduce the intake until they were able to stop completely.

With the help of the new doctor to alter the medication doses prescribed by the previous doctor, and with my support, they began executing my steps and guidance. This individual has managed to make a full turn around in life, leading a progressive and healthy lifestyle to this day. Note that I'm not saying to never take medication for depression, just be sure you trust your doctor enough and get more than one doctor's opinion before agreeing to take anything prescribed.

Gloria Anzaldua said *"Depression is useful. It signals that you need to make changes in your life, it challenges your tendency to withdraw, it reminds you to take action"*.

There Is Always Someone Who Cares!!!

There will be moments when you are at your lowest low, your mind will throw gas on the fire and play tricks on you. Leading you to believe that no one cares, that you're all alone in this world, and that everyone hates you!! I know, I've been there, luckily, I spotted the mind games and carved my way out.

When no one ask about us or enquire about our feelings, we take it as meaning they don't care about us. In reality many people are going through their own battles and may not wish, or have the capacity to indulge in enquiries of our feelings, but if you take a moment to ask for help and say how you feel, you will quickly realize that there are many people out there who care; it may not be the first person or the second person you talk to, but there will always be people who care.

If you are suffering from extreme depression and/or suicidal thoughts, please contact your local suicide hotline. Remember "If suicide ever crosses your mind, just know that I would rather listen to your story than attend your funeral."

Author unknown *"You feel lonely not when no one cares about you, but when someone you expect to care doesn't care about you at all".* Find who cares for you, not who you want to care for you.

Start Working On Your Passion.

As time progressed on my journey, I realized that one of the biggest positive impacts on my mental wellbeing was to focus on my passion. It could be finding your dream job, an interesting hobby, playing the sport you love the most, or as simple as just getting outside in nature. I have worked along with a handful of people in finding their passion/hobby, job/side hustle.

One of my biggest recollections is a family member who worked in a bank but was very unhappy through and through. Over the years he built up the courage to quit. Everyone thought he was crazy and not thinking straight, as this job was considered very secure and "paid highly". He went on to become a teacher and studied music. He then found the hobby of photography, where he has been taking phenomenal shots. As he grew in following his true desires and passion, he noticed significant transformation in his mental state that transitioned him to a place of mental peace.

Regarding me, I have opened multiple business and continue to build them from the ground up. I continue to mentor everyone around me who needs mentoring and if anyone battles this disease, I show them the path I took to be where I am today.

Delmas Ollivierre said *"Follow your dreams, you can't begin to imagine where it will take you"*.

Choose Your Music Wisely.

Like most things in life, when there is a positive reaction, there can also be an equal opposite (negative) reaction. When it comes to music, this can often move us and direct our feelings to different paths. Choosing the right type can guide us in either the right or wrong direction. I have nothing against any genre of music but against the words that some artist chose to sing about. I shuffle through different types of music based on the mood I'm in and have noticed that sometimes I would be in a very good, happy, jolly mood, then a song would come on with some negative lyrics and for one reason or another I would listen and not change the song. As the song plays on, my mood will gradually shift towards negative feelings, instigating negative trains of thoughts which would then lead me to selecting more negative choices of music to match the mood in which I was unwillingly placed in.

Going forward in life with the determination to not be defeated by depression, I choose my music very wisely. I love rap and hip hop but have removed songs with lyrics of negative messages, keeping songs with motivating messages and good quotes. I love country music, but I avoid ones with lyrics pertaining to bad memories such as the loss of a loved one or missing my horse lol. Instead, I focus more on up tempo or positive vibes.

Music plays a vital role in the way we feel, therefore, paying close attention to your selection can help you win more battles.

Gil Scott-Heron said "*Music has the power to make me feel good like nothing else does. It gives me some peace for a while. Takes me back to who I really am.*

Do As Much As You Can While You Can.

Times have changed for all of us, it's human nature to continue to outdo the generation before us and with great power comes great responsibility. The power we yield in this time is "INFORMATION and TECHNOLOGOY". Thanks to technology, information has become instant and readily available at our fingertips. With all the information out there, humans continue to develop more technology and more techniques for "tricking" the rest of the world. Mainly in return for money and power. I use the word trick based on that of a magician. As Bob Marley puts it "You can fool some people sometimes, but you can't fool all the people all the time."

Back in the day, getting information required a lot more work than it does today and the word convenient was not so "convenient" then. Today, if we are hungry, ordering food is a touch of a button, car repairs have become a touch of a button with mobile mechanics, any form of trade work required… you guessed it - a touch of a button! With these new apps, the world is at our fingertips. I'm saying all this to say; things have become so easily accessible that we don't even bother to try and learn anything new. We call "the guy" and then lounge around on our phones, most of the time being distracted by other people lives, when we can use that time to take the information readily available to us and better ourselves. **Prolong period of time scrolling through social media is also a very heavy hitter to the impact of depression we may face.** As the saying goes comparison is the thief of all joy! What does that mean you ask? Well, have you ever noticed that just about everyone who post stuff on social media only display their highlight moments? For example: they will display how much money they have/make, but never show the in-depth brutal work and sacrifice it takes to achieve it. They show beautiful pictures of where they are visiting around the world but never what they had to do to get there. Or even these highly rated "beautiful" (everyone is beautiful to me but I use the quotation as referral to media standard) models who post all these spectacular photos of themselves, but never the behind the scenes of how big the team is to hold the lights, the multiple angle shots taken until they get the most appealing one, the prolong time sitting in chairs having their makeup and hair done, and often, the length of time it takes to edit these photos just so they can have the perfect glare, perfect contrast. Now you are laying on your bed feeding your mind with all these highlighted moments of other peoples' lives. Then you find yourself getting lonely with your thoughts, wondering how all these people are "living their lives" while you seem to be caught up in a mediocre world. What you may not realize (which is obsoletely not your fault) is that some of these very lives that you may be looking at may be much more unhappy than you are, poorer than you are and even struggling highly with a depressive life. You may not see this because people have become very good at hiding the things they don't want the world to see, they have mastered that art of illusion (look at this hand of wonder as my other hand does the real "trick"). Moving forward I will advise you not to compare yourself with that of which you see in the world, because like the iceberg effect; there may be a lot more beneath the surface than what you can see.

    We have one life here to live. We should be doing all we can, while we can, and learning as much as we can, keeping our minds positively occupied. Do not compare your life with that of others, but instead, focus on constantly growing your knowledgebase which will help to keep you grounded and focused. This will lead to an enduring feeling of being progressive and purposeful which will in turn enrich you and elevate your mental and emotional wellbeing. LEARN ALL YOU CAN WHILE YOU CAN.

Beardsley Jones said, "*You have this one life. How do you want to spend it? Apologizing? Regretting? Questioning? Hating yourself? Dieting? Running after people who don't see you? Be brave. Believe in yourself. Do what feels good. Take risks. You have this one life. Make yourself proud*".

The Present Is A Gift.

Keeping your mind in check plays a role in keeping yourself calm and at peace. At the end of the day, we cannot stop the thoughts that come to us, but what we can do is control what we do with them. **If negative thoughts comes to mind,** we can choose to dwell on them and allow them to alter our mood negatively; or we can choose to treat them in our mind as birds in the sky: let the bird take its course, let it come and go leaving no trails in the sky, no emotions to dwell on.

I was born in St. Vincent and the Grenadines and migrated to Canada. Very often I found myself reminiscing on the life I left back in the "Land of my birth"; the hot sun, the year-round beach days, my family. These thoughts would usually take ahold of my emotions and send me down a "what if?" emotional drain, which would then take away from all the good that is right in front of me here in Canada. It wasn't until the year 2020 that I realized what a major toll these thoughts have taken on me over the years. I now avoid thinking of my past life at all costs as that trigger's depression, and I avoid trying to see into the future as this can trigger my anxiety. I must add here that I do not resent or hate my past life in any shape or form, as the past is what makes us who we are today, it's the thoughts of "what if" – What if I had stayed back on the island? What if I had kept my government job? What if I had not left my family and friends? - So, the issue is not my past, the issue is the "what ifs?" –Reminiscing on the paths not taken. Let go of what if and your mind will see you through.

Lao Tzu said: *"If you are depressed you are living in the past. If you are anxious you are living in the future. If you are at peace you are living in the present."*E

Exercise. Get Back To Nature

There is an old saying that goes "an idle mind is the devil's workshop." Which simply translate to a bored mind ponders unwanted thoughts. Sitting alone is a good way to get to know yourself but isolating for too long can create straying thoughts, which in most cases lead to negative trains of thought.

Isolating myself from the world always seems like the best idea in the moment of feeling depressed. Being locked in a room curled up in a ball somehow seems to create a false illusion that this "cocoon" will somehow protect me in one form or the other when in fact it does quite the opposite. I remember when I was younger without a care in the world, how much I loved hiking, riding my bike, sailing or even just being in the ocean floating peacefully with my eyes closed. With these thoughts, I remembered smiling while still in my "cocoon state" and asking myself "oh how nice would it be if I can do that stuff again?". Then I asked, "Why can't I? What is stopping me? NOTHING!" Then I got up and went outside for some fresh air as a start, then for a walk. Upon returning home, I felt a different mood, a different flow of energy. The next day, after battling with my thoughts again, I got up, got my bike, and went for a ride. Next day, a swim. The following day, a hike. Day after day, I kept hitting the outdoors and kept feeling better and better with more consistent periods of better, longer, happier days.

Then one day the rain came, and I'm not one of those who likes to dance in the rain, so while looking through the windowpane as the water trickled down, a deep state of depression started overtaking me again. As I sat there, my body kept feeling the urge of the routine, I wanted to go walking, swimming, riding, something, anything. Instead, I got down to the ground and started doing a few push-ups followed by a few sit ups and I felt my mental state get a lot calmer as my heart rate picked up. I continued to focus on doing different exercises and my state of depression subsided.

A body in motion tends to stay in motion. Exercise has many good physical and mental benefits, also, just being in nature creates calming effects on the mind. With these amazing benefits and effects, I will advise incorporating time out in nature as part of daily routines to create stronger peace of mind and a continuous relaxed state.

Anthony Douglas Williams said "Take a quiet walk with Mother Nature. It will nurture your mind, body, and soul."

Final thoughts.

My final thoughts to you are that of which I wish someone had told me in the midst of my darkest battle; Not every day will be perfect, but how we choose to react to situations is what will make the world of difference. Practice gratitude each day and appreciate the little things in life. Be mindful of the things you say to yourself for your subconscious mind takes each thought to heart.

Going to share with you what I always told "life" when I was feeling defeated. This always worked as a booster for me and got my mind back in the game

"Hey life……

How you doing life?.....

Tried to break me, huh life? You forgot God made me, huh life?....

Forgot I always shout "try me!" and not "why me?" huh life?...

The last stunt you pulled, you swore you finally broke me, huh life?....

Guess what life…..what?.... Now I'm stronger than ever, and this time I'm back to regain control of my life!

F.. depression, F… anxiety, We are the master of our own mind!!!

www.ingramcontent.com/pod-product-compliance
Lightning Source LLC
Chambersburg PA
CBHW050314220526
45465CB00005B/1993